Sunny's Sound Play

Hilary Lowe

J&R Press Ltd

To access the downloads that accompany this book use the following URL:
https://www.jr-press.co.uk/sunnys-sound-play-downloads.html

Introduction

Early babbling (experimental speech sound production) is a necessary precursor to speech development (Morris, 2010), and awareness of speech sounds (phonological awareness) is an important aspect of speech and literacy development (Hulme & Snowling, 2014). For children with speech sound disorders, intervention frequently includes speech sound awareness, discrimination, and production in play (Bowen, 2015).

This book aims to provide a fun way to help your child become more aware of speech sounds and how to make them. The sounds in the book cover a range of spoken consonants in the English language, including some which children usually find easy, and the most common ones which children with speech difficulties find hard. The sound-picture associations may be different to letter-sound schemes that your child will come across at nursery or school. This does not matter. The sound associations in this book are tried-and-tested ways which show your child how to say the sounds. The sounds are related to the noise that the object makes, not the initial letter of the word. This provides a firm foundation for speech and, later, literacy. Most of the sounds have an action to go with them which can be a useful extra prompt, but the exact actions are not critical to the sound production – you can make up your own, or use others that you know from other schemes if the sound association is the same. If you speak another language as well as English, you may like to make up sound associations for any additional sounds that occur in that language.

Use the book however it suits your child:

    To read at story-time

    For ideas of how to encourage babble during play

    To colour in.

Accompanying the book is a set of pictures to cut out for playing games with, and ideas of games to play.

Model the sounds yourself and let your child say or copy the sounds *if s/he wants to*. Encourage your child to look at you when you say the sounds. Some sounds are harder than others – praise good attempts! Even if the attempt is not quite right, you can still say "Good try!"

Ask your speech and language therapist to show you how to make the sounds. Use pure sounds (not the letter names):

Quiet, whispered sounds:	p, t, k, ch
Noisy sounds:	b, d, g
Long, quiet sounds:	f, s, sh
Long, noisy sounds:	v, z, w, l, y

If your child is interested, read the story/play the games often over the course of a few weeks. S/he is more likely to join in with the sounds after repetition and familiarity.

For a full list of the sounds see page 42.

References

Bowen, C. (2014) *Children's Speech Sound Disorders*. Chichester: Wiley-Blackwell.

Hulme, C. & Snowling, M. (2014) The interface between spoken and written language: Developmental disorders. *Philosophical Transactions of the Royal Society Biological Sciences*, 369(1634).

Morris, Sherrill R. (2010). Clinical application of the mean babbling level and syllable structure level. *Language, Speech & Hearing Services in Schools*, 41(2), 223–230.

Here is Sunny, my balloon.
It's a sunny afternoon.

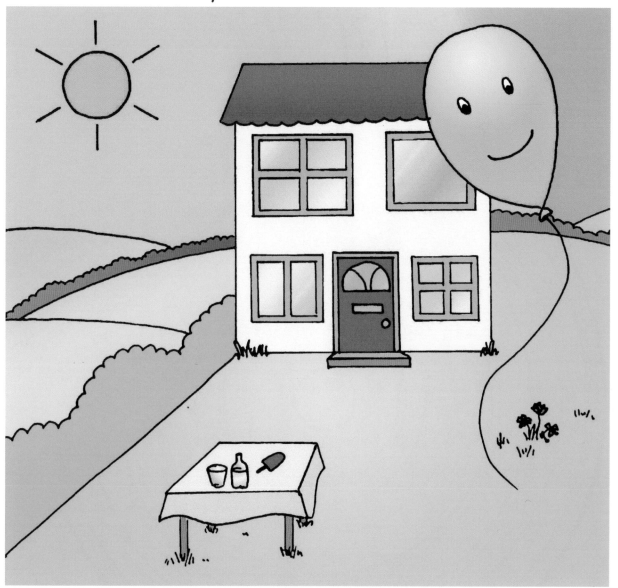

Sunny's floating through the sky.
What will he see as he goes by?

5

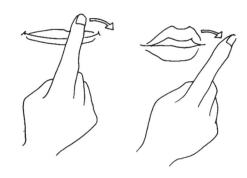

p – Lips together. A whispered sound.
Move finger as puff of air comes through
lips.

A candle on a birthday cake.

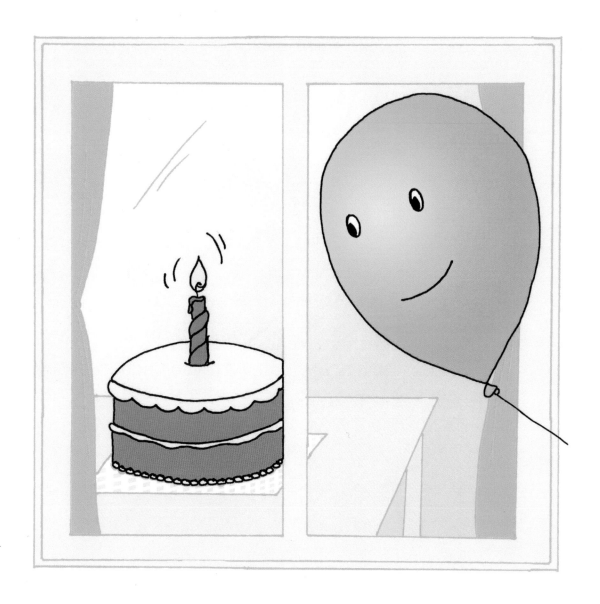

Sunny can blow the candle out with a **p**.
Can you?

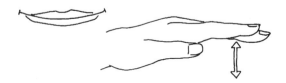

b – Lips together. A noisy sound.
Bounce an imaginary ball with your hand
as you say the sound.

What's that in the toy box?

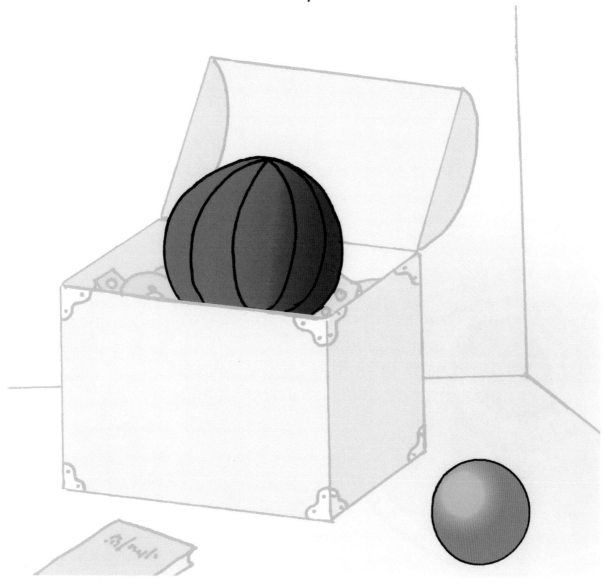

Bouncy ball says b – b – b.

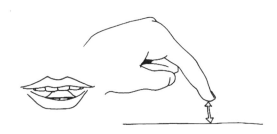

t – Tongue tip behind top teeth.
A whispered sound.
Tap finger in time with the sound to
indicate the drips of water coming out of
a tap.

Sunny can hear a tap dripping. Can you?

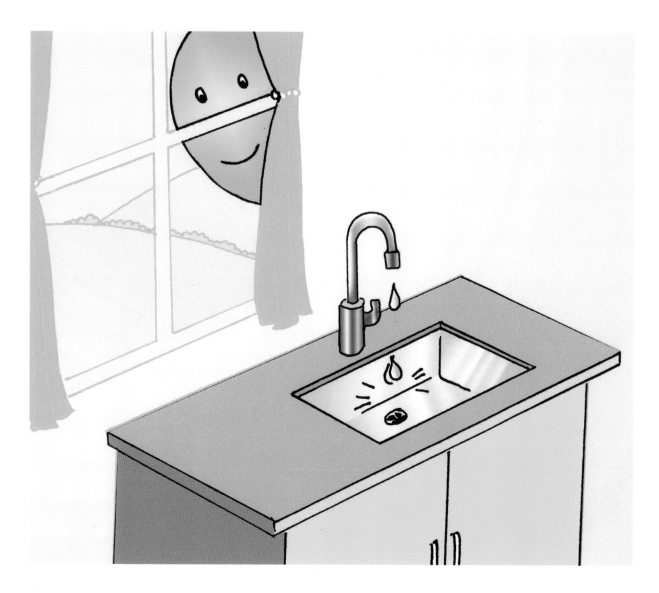

Dripping tap says † – † – †.

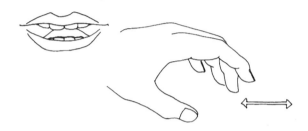

d - Tongue tip behind top teeth.
A noisy sound.
Mime moving along a toy tractor.

Sunny looks across the fields.
He can see a tractor.

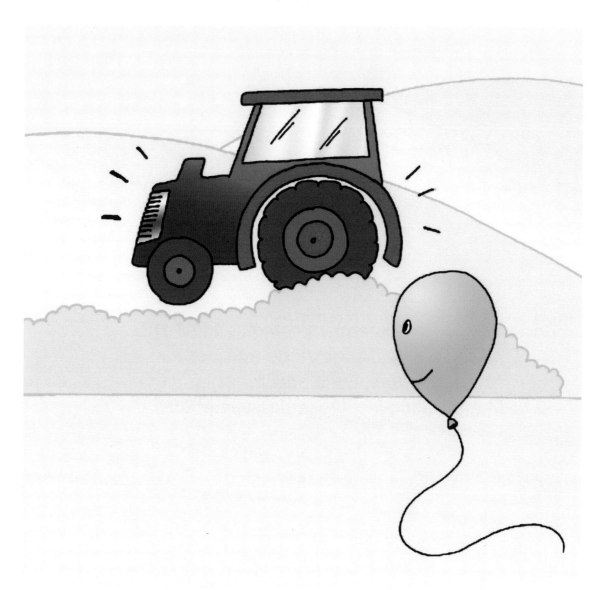

Noisy tractor goes **d – d – d – d – d**.

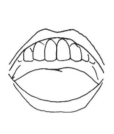 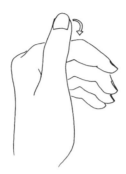

k – Mouth wide open, tongue up at the back (tongue tip down behind bottom teeth). A whispered sound.
Mime taking a picture on your phone.

Let's take a picture!

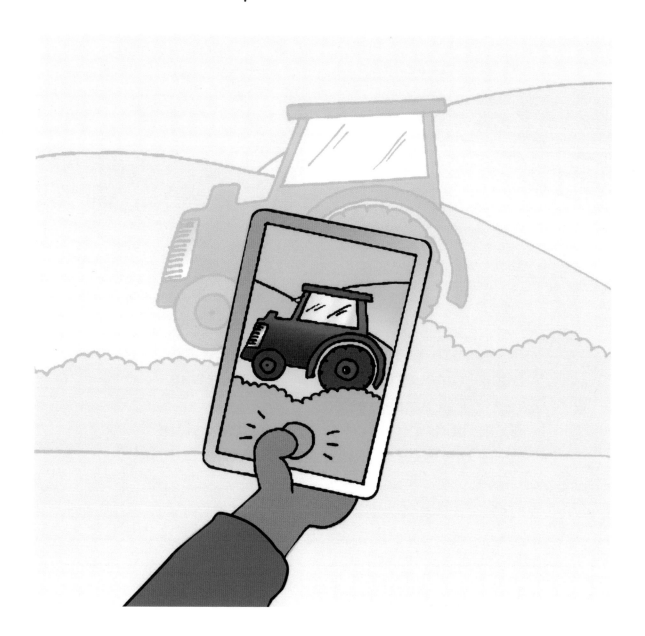

Camera clicks, **k**.

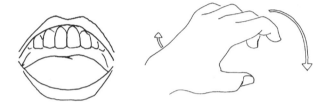

g – Mouth wide open, tongue up at the back (tongue tip down behind bottom teeth). A noisy sound.
Mime pouring juice from a bottle. The juice glugs as it comes out of the bottle!

Time for a snack. Biscuit to eat.
What's to drink?

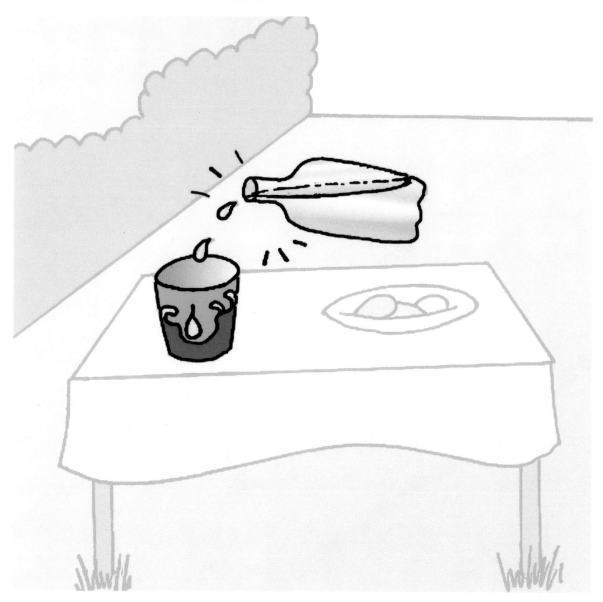

The bottle glugs g g g g g g.

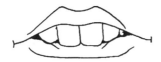

f – Top teeth on bottom lip. A long quiet sound.

Someone else wants a snack.

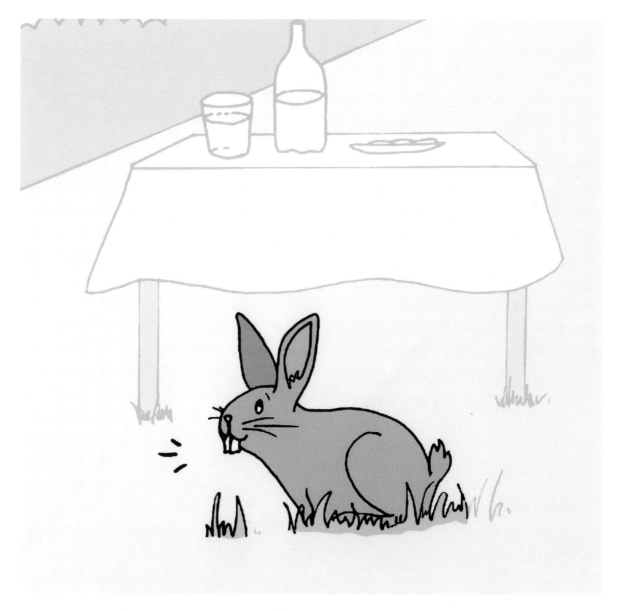

The rabbit's teeth are so big, that all he can say is fffff.......

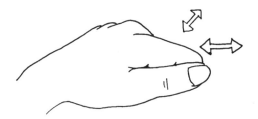

v – Top teeth on bottom lip.
A long noisy sound.
Mime moving the hoover back and forth.

Sunny can hear someone busy inside.

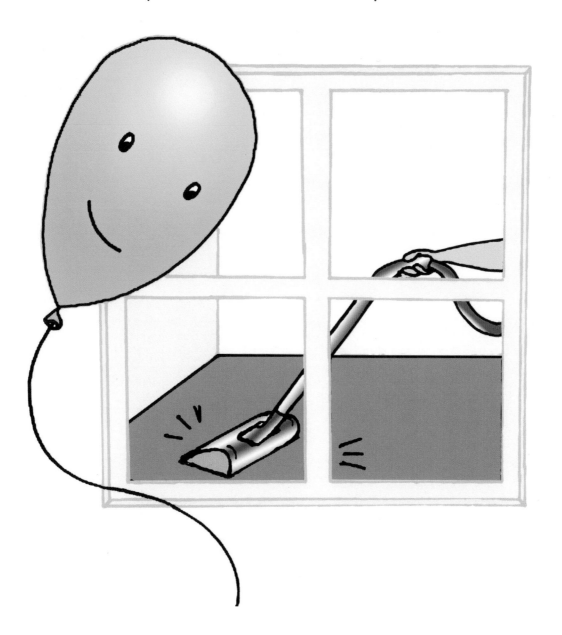

The hoover says vvvvv...

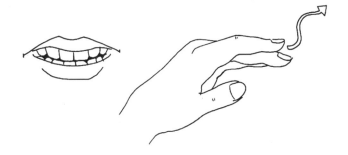

s –Teeth together. A long hissy sound.
Smile!
Mime a snake wiggling through the grass.

What's that in the long grass?

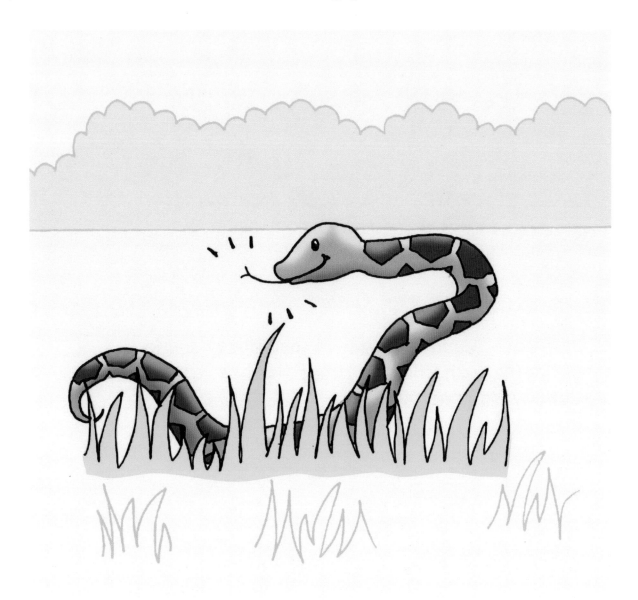

The snake hisses sssss...

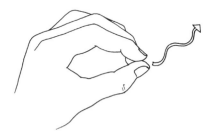

z – Teeth together. A long buzzy sound.
Make the flight path of the bee with
your fingertips.

And what's that in the flowers?

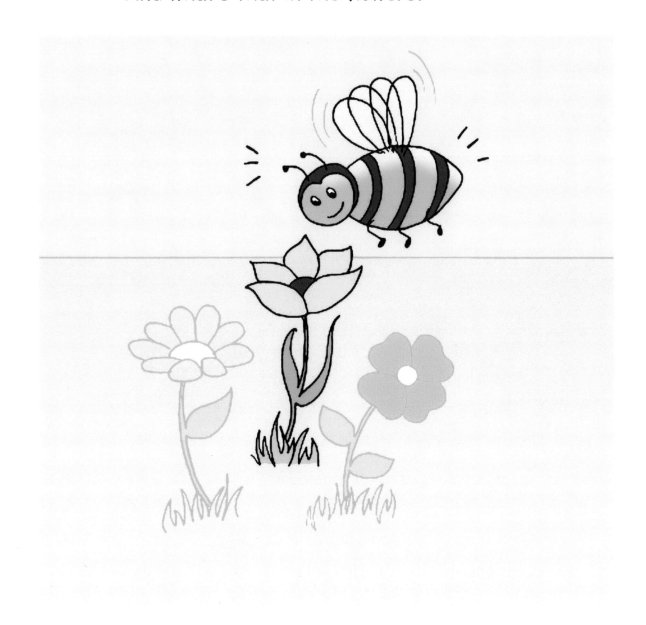

Buzzy bee says zzzzz...

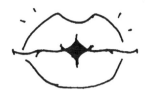

w – Make a little hole with your lips. It sounds like "oo" at the start.

Sunny can hear Dog barking.
Maybe he wants some supper.

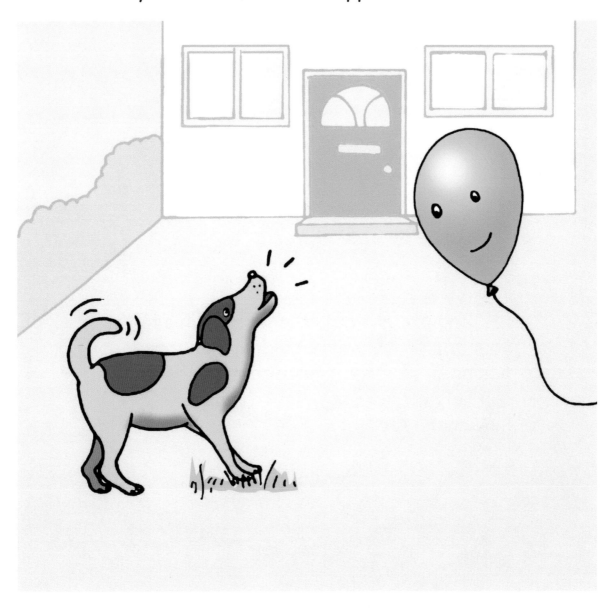

w – w – w!

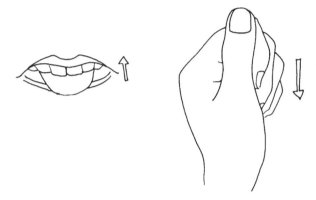

l – Tongue right out, then curl it in over your top teeth. Mime holding a lolly and licking it. This exaggerated movement will help achieve the right tongue movement for l.

A lollipop !?

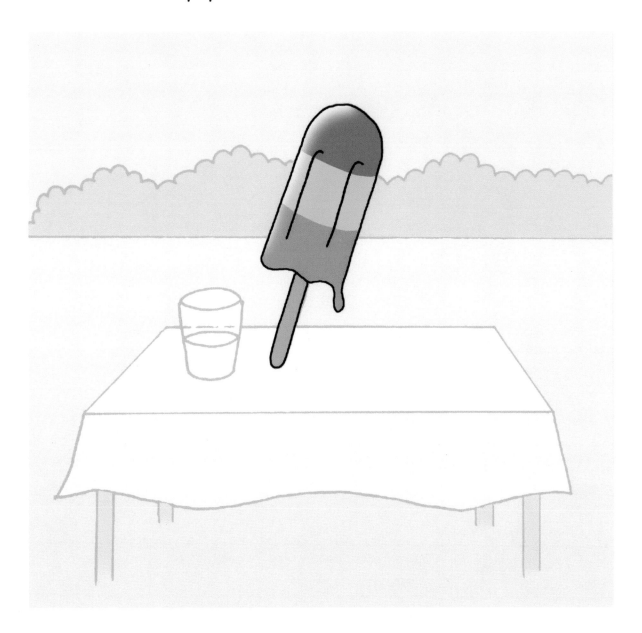

This is how you lick the lolly: l - l.

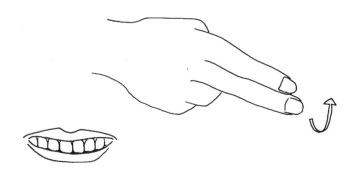

y – Smile! It sounds like "ee" to start with.
Make your fingers into a spoon and get a spoonful of yoghurt.

Dog is still hungry!
Can he have a yoghurt too?

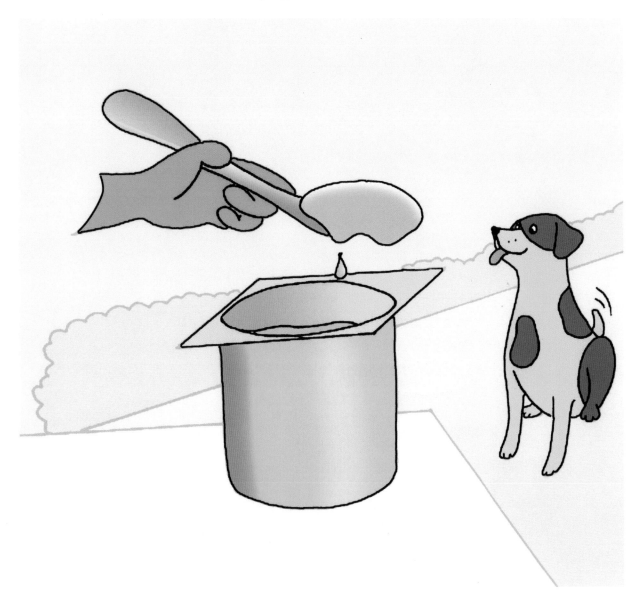

The yoghurt is yummy y – y.

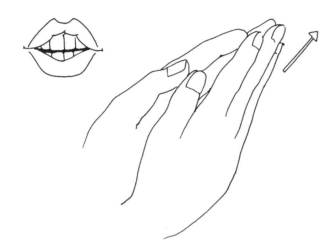

sh – Lips forward. A long hissy sound.
Make the shape of boat with your hands
and move it through the water.

Time for a bath.

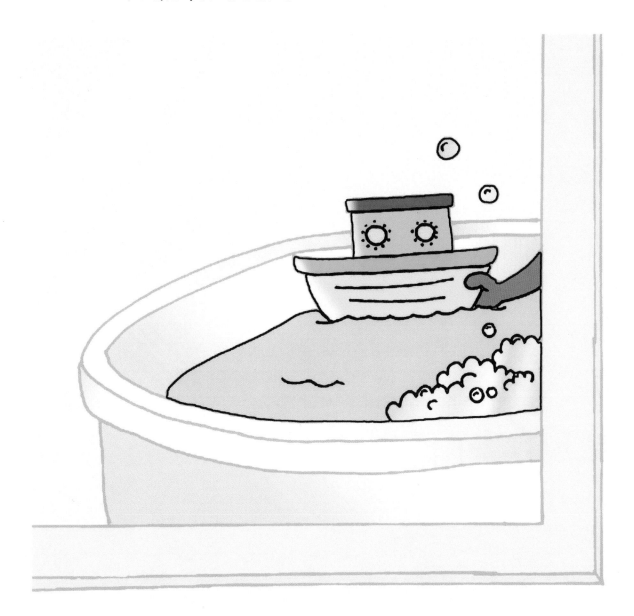

The boat goes through the water shh...

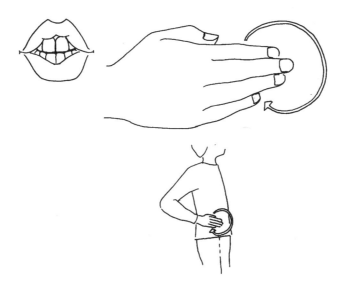

ch – Lips forward. Like sh but with a sharper start. Mime the wheels of the train going round by your side.

Are we allowed this in the bath?

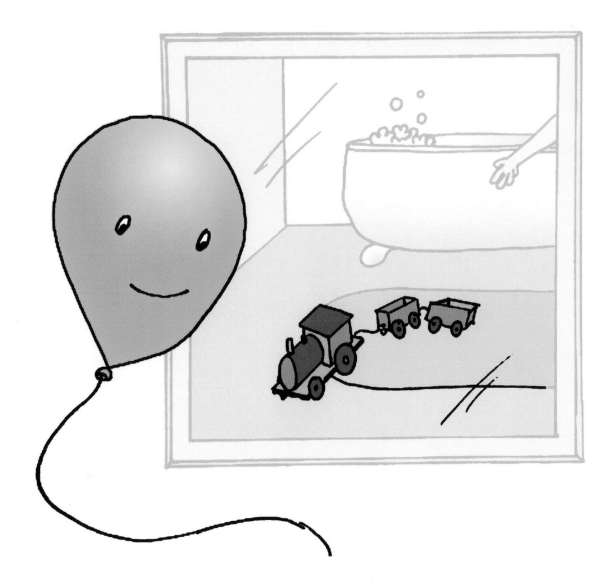

No! Off you go, train! Whoo - oo!
Ch – ch – ch – ch...

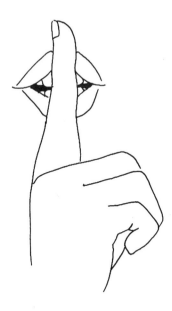

sh – Lips forward. Finger on lips.

Oh, where's Sunny?

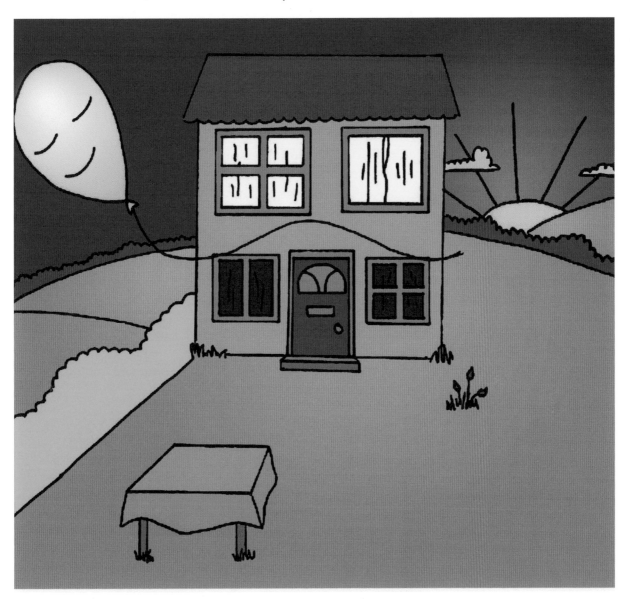

Floating away for another day.
Everyone's asleep! **Shh**...

Games to play with Sunny sounds

Association (getting to know the sound pictures). As you read the book and play the games, model the sounds *but don't make your child say them*. S/he will have a go if s/he want to. Praise any attempt with "good try!" It is important to keep your child's willingness to have a go even though they may not say the sounds accurately at the moment. You need two sets of picture cards (pages 40 and 41) to play these games. These are just suggestions – have fun making up your own games! You can also print the cards off by using this url: 000000000000000

- Pairs: Turn a set of no more than six pairs upside down. As you turn over two cards, say the sound. If you turn over two the same, you win the pair. Take turns. When it's your child's turn, s/he might say the sound if s/he wants to.

- Hang a set of sound pictures around the house - they will be a surprise when s/he finds them: "Well done – you've found 'p'!"

When your child knows which sound goes with which picture, s/he is ready to move on to discrimination.

Discrimination (listening to the difference between sounds). Prompt by showing the picture or doing the action, but move towards your child being able to choose the right sound picture by listening only.

Still *don't make your child say the sounds*. S/he will have a go if s/he wants to. Praise any attempt with "good try!" It is important to keep their willingness to have a go; their attempts will get better over time.

- Posting: make a post box out of an empty cereal packet. Spread up to six cards face up in front of the box. Say a sound: your child posts the right sound.

- Hide and find: Hide one set of the sounds round the room. Using the other set, turn up a card: say the sound: your child finds it. Give the action as a clue if necessary.

- Fishing for sounds: use a magnet on the end of a string for your fishing rod, and clip a paper clip to each picture. Spread the pictures out face up. Your child fishes for the sound you say.

- Pop-up-pirate: Place a sound under each dagger. Say a sound. Your child finds the sound you say and puts the dagger in. You can do this with other similar toys too.

When your child can listen and choose the right sound consistently, s/he is ready to move on to production.

Production (saying the sounds). Now, for all the discrimination games you have played, your child can take a turn at being the speaker and telling you which sound to post or to find. Praise any good attempt and move on. There will be other opportunities in the games to try again. If your child says the sound just right – say so! Use a mirror so that your child can see what their mouth is doing to make the sounds. You could also blu-tac a set of sound pictures around the bathroom mirror so that you can say one or two sounds together during teeth-cleaning time.

Have fun!

Erratum

The URL to be used to access the downloads is:
https://www.jr-press.co.uk/sunnys-sound-play-downloads.htm

This is also given on page 2 of this book

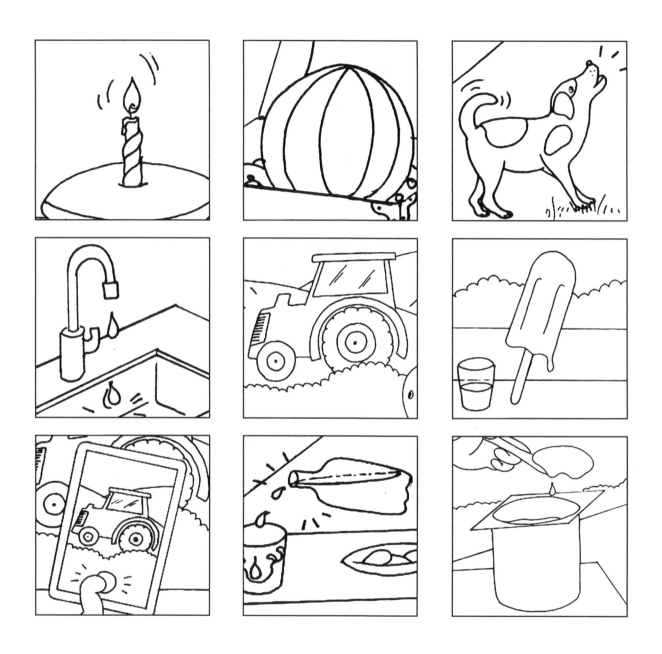

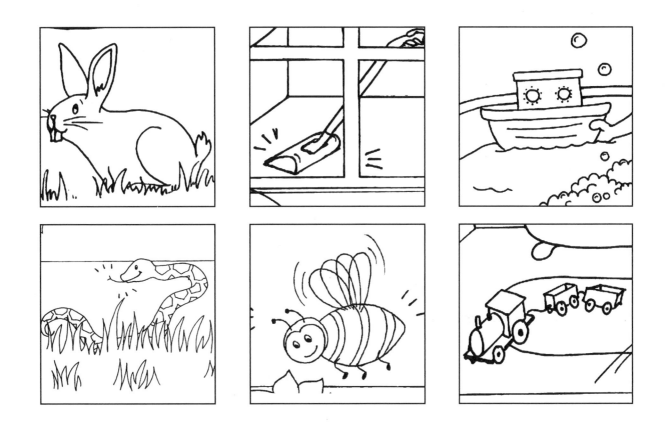

The Sounds